Banking With Your Liver
Why You Need To Stop Eating Cash

MICAH FRYE

DEDICATION

This work is dedicated to the concept of knowledge itself, our task to firmly grasp it, and the many people who swear they know something, but they don't. Also, to my wife Kathryn, my three kids: Natalie, Leo, and Audrey, my mom and dad Marci and David, my sister Jenna, her husband Jason, and the rest of my family and friends who have listened to my explanations.

CONTENTS

DISCLAIMER

The content of this book is for informational purposes only and is <u>not intended</u> to replace consultation with a licensed primary care physician. The author strongly recommends that you consult with your own licensed healthcare practitioner regarding the implementation of any of the recommendations made in this book <u>before</u> undertaking any nutritional or fitness program. If you do engage in the implementation of any of the recommendations made in this book, then you agree that you do so at your own risk, are consensually and voluntarily participating in those activities, assume all risk of injury to yourself, and you agree to release and discharge the author from any and all claims or causes of action, known or unknown, arising out of the contents of this book. The use of this book implies your acceptance of this disclaimer.

CHAPTER 1
WHO IS YOUR LIVER?

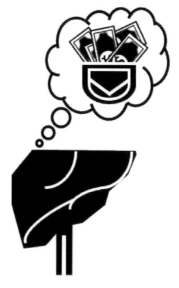

Your liver is the organ that adds fat to and removes fat from your body, so it's the focus of the book. Also, your liver sends energy to the other organs and requires energy itself, so your liver's obsession with energy is another focus of the book [1].

For your liver, **energy is money** that your liver uses to "pay" and fuel the other organs, itself, and its abundant **savings account (your stored body fat)**.

Your goal though, is to somehow force your liver to **withdraw from its savings account (burn your stored body fat)**. Throughout the day, you provide income to your liver by eating different types of money and your liver carefully decides how that income gets used and how your body looks and functions.

CHAPTER 2
YOUR LIVER'S POCKET CASH

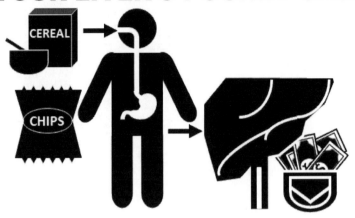

Your income choices are being directed by your money hungry liver who craves cash in its pockets. **Dietary carbohydrates are your liver's cash and glycogen stores (stored carbs) are your liver's pockets** [1]. If you regularly consume carbohydrates, your liver uses that cash to overfill its pockets and puts the extra bills directly into its savings account. **Stored fat around the body is the liver's savings account and lipogenesis is how your liver easily puts its pocket cash directly into its savings account** [2, 20]. Yes, the stored fat around your body is from the surplus of dietary carbohydrates you're consuming [20].

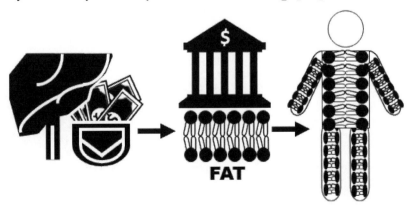

If you continue to regularly eat cash (carbs), then your liver's pockets (glycogen stores) will always remain stuffed, and your liver won't ever attempt to withdraw from its savings account (your stored fat). Whether it's a sweet carbohydrate (simple) or a not sweet carbohydrate (complex), it's all cash for your liver's pockets [see Figure 1]. **Why would your liver withdraw from its savings account when you keep filling its pockets with cash?**

Your liver's pocket cash (stored carbs) is its most immediate obsession and anytime you've felt hungry, your liver has been signaling your stomach to send you notifications that the liver's pocket cash (storage of carbs) is running low. **The hunger hormone ghrelin**, produced by the stomach, **is the notification of a low cash balance** [3]. For cash eaters (carb eaters), this hunger is intense because of how panicked their liver is without cash (stored carbs) on hand. However, there is a much better source of income that's worth more, is used cleanly and efficiently, reduces the hunger notifications, and allows your liver to start banking instead of relying on cash for everything.

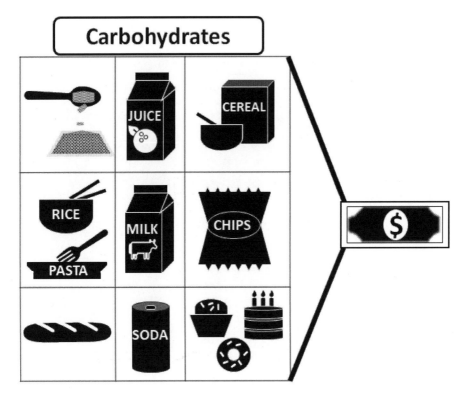

[Figure 1]

CHAPTER 3
YOUR LIVER'S CHECKING ACCOUNT

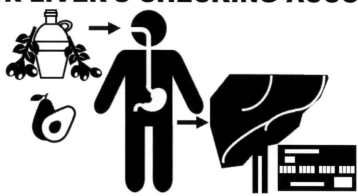

For the same reasons you don't need cash in real life, your liver does not need any dietary carbohydrates [4]. In fact, in real life, you can go your whole day buying essentials without using any cash at all. If you're anything like me, you have a checking account and you probably just use your check/debit card for all your purchases. Your liver can and should do the exact same thing.

Dietary fats are your liver's checking account [see Figure 2]. If you do continue to eat cash (dietary carbs), your liver does not see a reason to access its checking account (dietary fat) for money (energy) because there's so much cash (stored carb) in its pockets (glycogen stores); its checking account (dietary fat) is largely ignored.

Therefore, when your liver's pockets get low and you feel hungry, **don't eat cash ever (0g carb/day)**, and instead put money directly into your liver's checking account by **eating**

good fats, lean proteins, and dark leafy green micronutrients (the logo of the book).

Advisory Lifetime cash (carb) eaters look here. When you completely stop eating cash (dietary carbs) for the first time (0g carb/day), your liver's pockets (glycogen stores) will be depleted, and your liver and your brain will not be happy about it. They've been running on cash (dietary carbs) their whole lives, and you've just taken away the very thing that sustains their being! During this time, your liver starts to scramble for cash (carbs), and you receive intense notifications of low cash balance in the form of hunger pangs, nausea, fatigue, dizziness, headaches, and flu-like symptoms. **This carb/keto flu is your liver's transition from only using cash (dietary carbs) to exclusively banking with its checking account (using dietary fat)** [5].

Yes, the symptoms that come with getting your liver off cash (dietary carbs) are not fun, but it's helpful to know that during this temporary transition, nothing's actually wrong with you; it just sucks. **The "cash flu" (carb flu) is essentially a set of temporary false symptoms** that amount to your liver and your brain stomping their feet because they didn't get their dose of cash (carbs). You're not actually sick!

This transition will last anywhere from 3 to 7 days **if you maintain 0g carb/day**, but this time is made exponentially easier and shorter by eating **good fats, lean proteins, and dark leafy green micronutrients** (the logo of the book). If you can get all your protein and all your micronutrients paired with a healthy fat during this transition period, then your liver and brain will quietly calm down and realize there's tons of money (energy) in the liver's checking account (dietary fat).

Post transition, your liver must regularly use the checking account (dietary fat) for its money (energy) needs; it must start banking. It's at this point that your liver receives its own **check card** containing the balance of **its checking account, the fats you're eating**. Now the liver can pay the organs directly with the check card. **Ketones**, produced from breaking down dietary fats, are how your liver uses its **check card to pay and fuel the other organs directly** [1,8].

What's nice is that the check card is worth more than cash. **Fat is 9 calories/gram while carbohydrates are 4 calories/gram**, so your liver and the other organs will all prefer using the check card (dietary fat) instead of cash (dietary carbs) because of its greater value. This more efficient money also improves organ performance, provides satiety, enhances the brain's functions, and preserves muscle [6]. Using the check card (dietary fat) is so much better than using cash (dietary carbs), and your liver, brain, and muscles all agree.

There is one problem, however. The liver's pockets, the muscles' pockets, and a small portion of the brain only accept cash. If only there were a way for the liver to get cash using the check card…

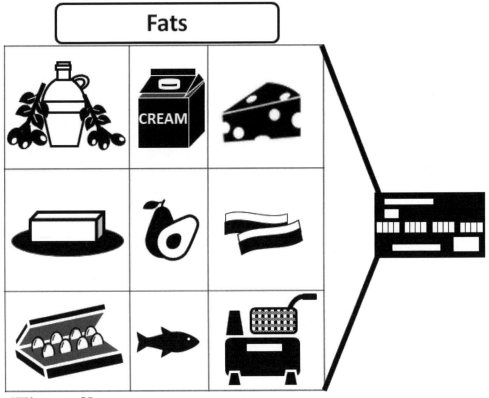

[Figure 2]

CHAPTER 4
YOUR LIVER'S ATM

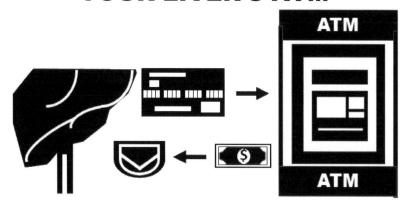

Once your liver has a check card, it needs to know how to get cash for those organs that simply won't accept card payments. Fortunately, the liver has an ATM, and the liver can use its check card to withdraw cash from the checking account at the ATM. **Gluconeogenesis is your liver's ATM, and it allows your liver to convert fat into glucose** (fat→sugar) [7]. You may be wondering why glucose hasn't been mentioned yet in a book about diet and nutrition, but the omission was intentional.

One intention of this book is to break the association we all instinctually make between glucose needed by the body and dietary carbohydrates. **Dietary carbohydrates are not essential** for creating glucose in your body [4]! All glucose (pocket cash) needed by your liver and muscles **can and should be produced by gluconeogenesis** instead of dietary carbohydrates.

In other words, if your liver wants cash (glucose), then it

should just go to the ATM (gluconeogenesis) and get the cash itself. Your liver can use this withdrawn cash (glucose) to pay those cash only organs and its own pockets (glycogen stores). When your liver no longer has a pocket cash income (dietary carbohydrates) and is using the ATM (gluconeogenesis) regularly, congratulations! Your liver is banking. Now, you need to bank along with your liver.

CHAPTER 5
YOUR LIVER'S SAVINGS ACCOUNT

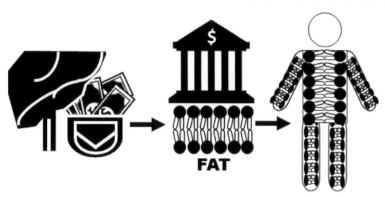

Before your liver ever gets into regular banking, it takes all the extra cash (stored carbs) bursting from its pockets dumps a pile of it on the bank teller's desk and demands that the teller deposit it into your liver's **savings account (your stored fat)** via lipogenesis (carb→fat). But after your liver has a check card and is fully banking and using the ATM as needed, **the savings account (your stored fat) can become a source of income** [8]!

Just like your liver can access the ATM to withdraw cash from its checking account, your liver can access the ATM (gluconeogenesis) to **withdraw cash from its savings account** [7]. Your liver will convert your stored fat into glucose (pocket cash) as well as break down your stored fat for direct energy from ketones (check card) …that's how you lose fat!

Here's the tricky part. **How do you force your liver to withdraw from its savings?** Well, to force your liver to withdraw from its checking account, you had to **deplete its pocket cash**. So, to force your liver to withdraw from its savings account, you'll have to **deplete its checking account** as well.

Depleting your liver's checking account requires you to withhold income from your liver. **Fasting is withholding income from your liver**. The liver still spends money (energy) to pay (fuel) all your organs while you're withholding income (fasting), so the liver must access money (energy) from somewhere; good thing it has bank accounts.

The traditional problem that most people run into with fasting is that their livers are still reliant on cash (dietary carbs) and aren't banking at all, so when the liver's pockets get low from withholding income, there's **no check card (ketones) or ATM (gluconeogenesis)** to meet the liver's needs. The cash eater's liver begins to panic and gets the stomach to send intense notifications of a low balance in the form of hunger pangs, nausea, and headaches, and likely most cash eaters will stop fasting because of how brutal and ineffective it is; **withholding income is not for cash (carb) eaters**.

However, if your liver is consistently banking **without any cash income (0g carb/day)** and visiting the ATM regularly, then withholding income (fasting) becomes much easier and beneficial for you. You will still feel hungry, but the hunger pangs become short lived, mild, or nonexistent.

Your extended fast should *always* be preceded by a healthy day of **eating good fats, lean proteins, and dark leafy green micronutrients** (the logo of the book). If you can reach your protein total and absorb all your micronutrients with healthy fats by your last meal, then from there you can fast or **withhold income for up to 24 hours** safely and with little effort.

You can decide the duration and frequency of fasting that you can handle as long as you precede the fast with the **recommended daily income for your liver** [see Chapter 7].

During this time of withholding income (fasting), your liver's checking account (dietary fat) will quickly deplete and, by about 15 hours after your last meal, your liver will be forced to **withdraw from its savings account at the ATM** (stored fat gluconeogenesis) or transfer money from the savings to the checking and use the check card directly (stored fat ketones). Past hour 16, your liver is withdrawing from its savings (your stored fat) at an exponential rate [9].

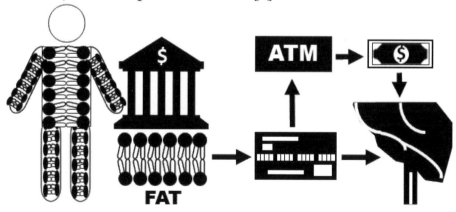

Congratulations! That's losing real weight. You must get your liver to **withdraw from its savings account to lose body fat,**

but your liver needs to be regularly using the check card (ketones) and void of pocket cash (dietary carbs) to allow you to withhold income (fast) and force your liver to spend its money (energy) safely and effectively.

This is how banking with your liver should be. You control when your liver uses its savings account by withholding its checking account income. No need to eat cash. Ever.

CHAPTER 6
YOUR LIVER'S PROPERTY

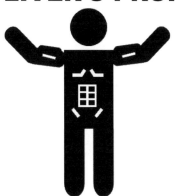

Along with obsessing over money (energy), your liver has the responsibility to help construct and preserve property. **Muscles are your liver's property** and property requires construction materials.

Protein is your liver's construction material for property [see Figure 3]. Your liver has to make sure that each property (muscle) gets enough construction material (protein) to preserve existing property (muscle) or to construct more property (muscle) if needed.

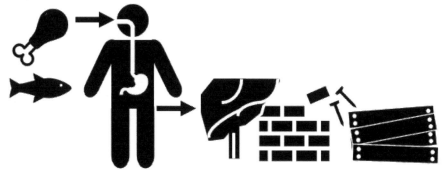

There's a problem though. The liver is not allowed to use construction materials (protein) on property (muscles) without the proper permits. **Micronutrients are your liver's construction permits, and they allow your liver to put protein into your muscles** [see Figure 4].

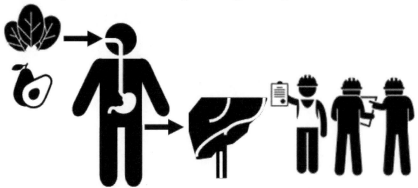

Without eating dark leafy green micronutrients, the protein you eat does not enter the muscle; property cannot be built [10]. Any consumed protein that didn't enter the muscles will be converted to glucose, in other words, the liver liquidates the **unused construction material (glucogenic amino acids)** for cash.

You can avoid construction material liquidation by eating a combination of **construction permits (dark leafy green micronutrients)** and **construction materials (protein)** every day.

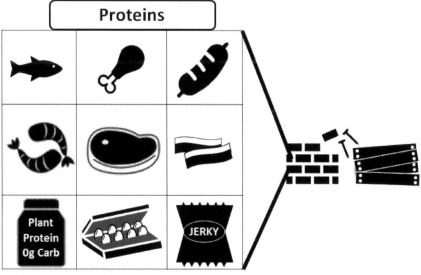

[Figure 3]

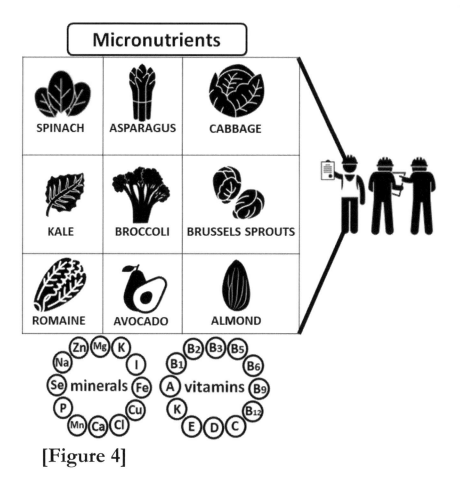

[Figure 4]

CHAPTER 7
YOUR LIVER'S RECOMMENDED DAILY INCOME

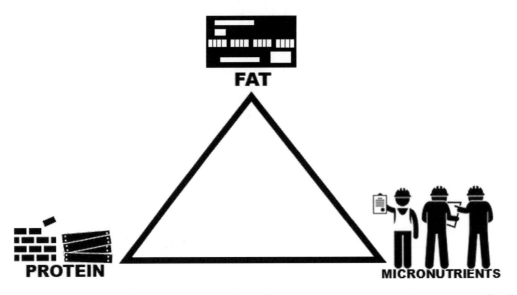

In most diet books, there's all this counting of unspecified calories, random times of day to eat things, and arbitrary point systems that do nothing; it's all a bunch of garbage. **Your diet is your liver's daily income** and it's the type of money in the income that matters. So, here is the **recommended daily income** if you are banking with your liver at **0g carb/day**.

1. Eat 1g of **protein** per pound of lean body mass per day.
2. Eat the **fat** that comes with your protein.
3. Eat 3-5 cups of raw **dark leafy greens** per day.
4. Pair healthy fats like **avocado** and **olive oil** with your greens.

That's it. There is no calorie allotment, there's no timing, and there's no stupid point system. If you get hungry, eat more. If you want to lose more stored fat, withhold income (fast) for a day after consuming a day's income. Simplest diet ever.

The only real numerical requirement is the protein total and **even if you're not trying to gain muscle, you need to protect the muscle you already have** with enough construction materials (protein) and permits (micronutrients). So, <u>everyone must always get at least 1g of protein per pound of lean body mass per day</u> to avoid muscle loss whether you're male, female, athletic, nonathletic, or otherwise [21].

If your lean body mass is 120 lbs., then you need to eat 120g of protein per day to preserve it. Ask your doctor for your lean body mass or use an online lean body mass estimator. **Your lean body mass in pounds is your daily protein total in grams**.

If you do wish to gain muscle, simply make your daily protein total equal to the lean body mass you desire. For example, if someone has a lean body mass of 120 lbs., but desires to have a lean body mass of 130 lbs. to add more muscle to their frame, they will eat 130g of protein per day.

The best proteins are fish and seafood like salmon and shrimp, because they're no carb, high protein, and good fat. Other good proteins include chicken, eggs, turkey, beef, pork, and 0g carb plant protein powders/shakes. No breaded or sugared proteins ever!

The best fats are fish fats, olive oil, and avocado because they're high in anti-inflammatory fatty acids that keep your liver burning fat cleanly. Other good fats include chicken fat, beef fat, egg yolk, and almond fat.

The best micronutrients, without any question, are spinach and avocado because together they contain every micronutrient you'll ever need. Other good micronutrients include kale, broccoli, and romaine, but it's most important to look for any dark leafy green and get at least 3-5 cups per day.

Also, many of the **dark leafy green micronutrients** cannot be absorbed by your body unless they are **consumed with a fat**, so the recommended daily income has you pairing an **avocado or olive oil** with your dark leafy green micronutrients.

You might be thinking that the recommended daily income has...cash (carbs)! Look, dark leafy green plants have carbohydrates in them because they photosynthesize, so spinach and avocado both have **trace amounts of cash (carbs)**. But these carbs amount to pennies on the dollar, and when you're banking with your liver, pennies from construction permits don't count. You do not need to count the 1g net carb in spinach or the 2.5g net carbs in avocado…it's still no carb.

By accurately using this recommended daily income, your liver can satisfy its money (energy) needs with its checking (dietary fat) or savings account (your stored body fat) and maintain or construct property (muscle) with its construction materials (protein) and permits (micronutrients).

CHAPTER 8
YOUR LIVER'S SPENDING

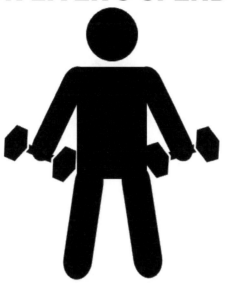

All the activities your organs do cost your liver money (energy). How much money each organ costs to run varies from person to person. **Your resting metabolic rate (RMR) is the total money each of your organs costs your liver to run in a day** [11]. This number, your RMR, is your liver's biggest expense during the day, but there of course is another expense...

Presumably, you don't lie in bed for 24 hours, so any moving you do beyond inhaling oxygen and exhaling CO_2 will be another expense for your liver. **The exercising of your muscles is your liver's second biggest expense and the liver's signal to put construction materials into property to preserve and repair.** Muscles cost a lot to move around because they also have pockets (glycogen stores) that require cash (glucose), so during exercise, your banking literate liver is visiting the ATM (gluconeogenesis) a lot when your muscles' pockets get low. You want your liver spending its income, so this is perfect.

To capitalize on this spending, you need simplistic efficient exercises that require resistance training. **Using free weights provides resistance**. *Read Disclaimer*

To choose the correct weight, pick up two equal free weights (at a gym or fitness store) and hold your arms straight out to the left and right, the **"iron cross"**.

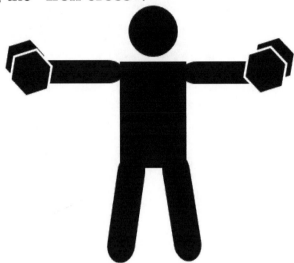

If the **iron cross** is too easy, go heavier. If you can't even do it, go lighter. You want to select the weight that allows you to just **barely do the iron cross**. Once you select that weight, it's time to get some property moving.

The most expensive property in the body is located in the thigh-butt neighborhood, so start by holding your free weights at your sides and doing **30 squats**.

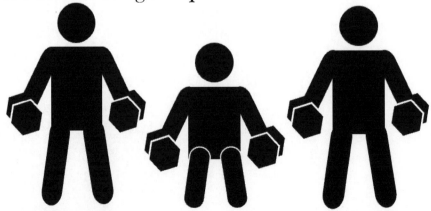

Then take your free weights and do **30 flies** (some people call them wing flappers, lol).

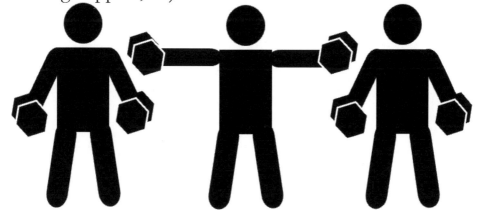

Then take your free weights and do **30 curls to presses**.

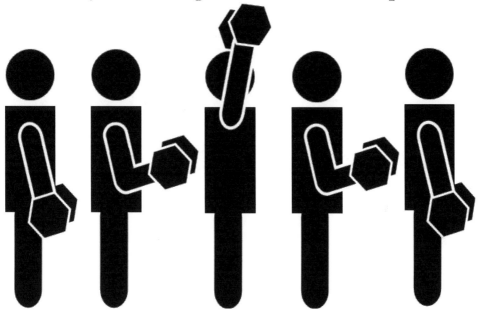

You also want to get your **abdominal property** (abs) moving to ensure better posture, lifting form, and overall strength. Start by lying on your back on the ground and extending your legs with your arms extended above your head. Try to keep your legs extended **without touching the ground with about an inch of clearance** between your ankles and the ground. Do the same thing with the back of your head and your extended arms.

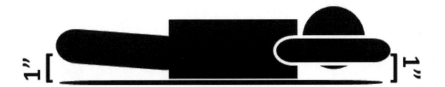

Once in proper **leg lift form**, bring your extended legs and your extended arms together and return them to an inch above the ground. **Do 30 leg lift crunches.**

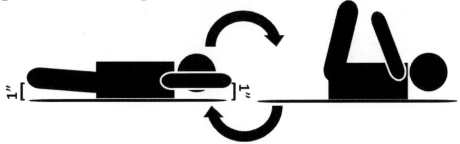

Then from leg lift form, spread your extended legs and spread your extended arms and assume the **starfish position**.

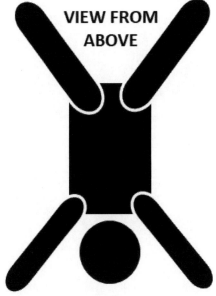

Bring your extended left leg to your extended right arm, return to **starfish** position, and then bring your extended right leg to your extended left arm and return to **starfish** position. **Do 30 starfishes.**

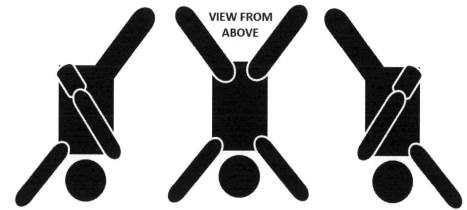

Then return to **leg lift form**. The last abdominal exercise is the **ladder climb**. Bend your extended left leg and bring your left knee in to your chest while keeping your right leg extended and off the ground. Then touch your left knee with your right elbow and return to leg lift form. Do the same thing with the right knee and left elbow. **Do 30 ladder climbs**.

VIEW FROM
ABOVE

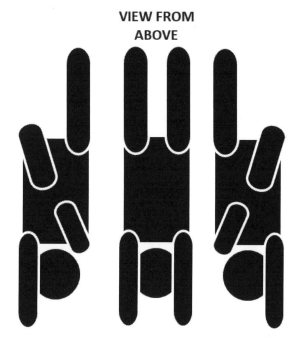

You can also exercise your muscles by powerwalking/jogging up **inclines**. When you're on a treadmill, put the **treadmill to its highest incline** and find the speed (slow is fine) you could go up that incline for 15 minutes, **without holding the bars**. When you find cement or industrial grade stairs (usually outside), jog up and down those stairs for 15 minutes. When you find natural hills outside, **powerwalk or jog up** the hill and **powerwalk down** the hill for 15 minutes.

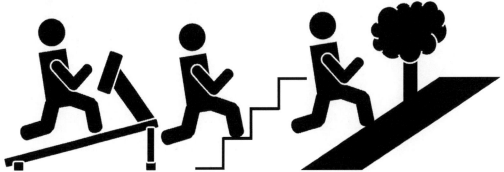

Doing these exercises forces the liver to spend money on the muscles in addition to all the other organs the liver has to pay. Including the adequate amount of resistance training tells your liver that your muscles are worthy of preservation. In summary, for 2-3 times a week:

1. Find your **iron cross weight** in a pair of free weights.
2. Do **30 squats, 30 flies**, and **30 curls to presses**.
3. Lie in **leg lift position**.
4. Do **30 leg lift crunches, 30 starfishes**, and **30 ladder climbs**.
5. Find an incline.
6. **Powerwalk or jog up** the incline and **powerwalk down** the incline for at least **15 minutes**.
   Do not go <u>down</u> an incline on a treadmill

CHAPTER 9
THE CASE AGAINST CASH

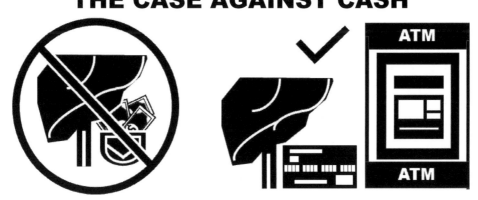

Dietary carbohydrates (cash in this book) are not essential and are detrimental to your health. There exists no function exclusive to dietary carbohydrates that cannot be achieved directly or indirectly with fat, protein, and micronutrients. None. There do exist however, several side effects exclusive to dietary carbohydrates that are prevented by consuming fat, protein, and micronutrients. Several.

We teach our youth that our bodies need glucose for energy and glucose is a carbohydrate. These are true facts. What we don't teach our youth is that our bodies need glucose **and glucose can be created from fat without any dietary carbohydrates ever needed!**

Very few people then have been taught about and have retained the idea of **gluconeogenesis (fat→sugar), the liver's ATM**. Yet the average person will readily tell you that "you have to eat carbs for energy." Would these people still think that "you have to eat carbs for energy" if they knew their livers could efficiently convert fat into glucose? Why don't most people know about **the liver's ATM**? (btw the kidneys have an ATM too)

Well, it's that pesky transition period when your liver's getting off cash (dietary carbs) and into using the checking account (dietary fat), **the cash/carb flu**. You see, cash eaters think that avoiding carbs leaves you in this flu-like state forever because every time the average cash eater tries to stop eating carbs, they start to feel like crap. The lifelong cash eater then associates no carb with feeling sick, never achieves 0g carb/day, and never rides out the **temporary** carb flu to achieve the benefits of no carb; their livers don't ever start banking.

The cash eater just can't understand that **the cash flu is a set of temporary false symptoms**. Couple this with the knee jerk fact spew, "carbs are for energy," and people firmly believe that the temporary carb flu is a permanent state of starvation that makes you sick and tired forever. It's absolute nonsense!

Pro-cash dieticians, nearly always lifelong cash eaters themselves, will have you believe that **the liver's ATM, gluconeogenesis**, is therefore a starvation process to be avoided by…eating more carbs…ugh.

But you know from reading the chapter called, "Your Liver's ATM" that if you never eat carbs (0g carb/day) and instead consume good fats, lean proteins, and dark leafy green micronutrients, then your liver is using **gluconeogenesis** safely and efficiently to **replace ANY function of dietary carbohydrates** and by no means are you starving!

Dietary carbohydrates are therefore not essential because of gluconeogenesis and the fact that fat is a superior source of energy to carbs. The liver does not need a cash income because it has an ATM and more money in its checking and savings accounts.

Along with not being essential, **dietary carbohydrates are detrimental** to your health. They are responsible for a whole host of **problems and conditions including the 5 "I"s**:

- Inflammation [12, 19]
- Injury [13]
- Illness [14, 18]
- Insulin spikes [14]
- Irregular blood sugar [15]

By consuming carbohydrates, you can expect more water under your skin, fat under your skin, water in your muscles, fat in your muscles, bloating, pain from trauma, swelling when injured, exhaustion from exercise, hunger, and total weight gain.

Carbohydrates make you hold on to so much water because each gram of carbohydrate holds about 3 grams of water inside of you. Carbohydrates make you store so much fat because they are what your liver converts into stored fat around the body.

Carbohydrates make you swell because of the increased inflammation they are causing in your skeletal muscle. Carbohydrates make you tired because they stop your liver from accessing fat in times of caloric deficit during exercise. Carbohydrates make you gain weight because of all the swelling, retained water, exhaustion, and stored fat.

The case against cash, dietary carbohydrates, is clear. **Why would you eat something that's not essential and causes you to retain water and swell up?**

CHAPTER 10
NUTRITION MYTHS DEBUNKED

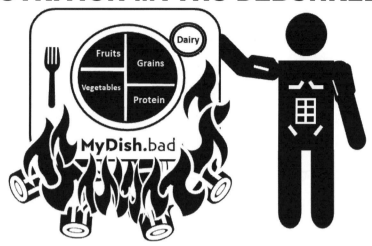

Myth #1 – Dietary carbohydrates are essential.

Fact #1 – **Your liver can synthesize its own glucose** from dietary fat via **gluconeogenesis**.

Your liver can access the ATM to get its pocket cash. So can your kidneys.

Myth #2 – Calorie deficits are bad for you.

Fact #2 – Calorie deficits are **bad for carbohydrate eaters**. People who eat 0g carbs/day, good fats, lean proteins, and micronutrients can go into calorie deficits just fine. Withholding income is bad for cash eaters. People who eat for the liver's checking account can withhold income just fine.

Myth #3 – Fasting leads to muscle loss.

Fact #3 – Fasting leads to muscle loss for carbohydrate eaters. **People who eat good fats, lean proteins, and micronutrients can fast without any muscle loss**. For cash (carb) eaters, withholding income (fasting) leads to the liver liquidating property (muscle) for cash (glucose). For people banking with their livers, withholding income leads to the liver withdrawing from its savings account (your stored fat) for cash (glucose) and using construction materials (protein) and permits (micronutrients) to preserve property (muscles).

Myth #4 – Low carb diets lead to heart disease.

Fact #4 – **Low carb diets that neither distinguish between good fats and bad fats nor recommend daily protein and micronutrient totals can lead to heart disease**.

Myth #5 – You can't lose fat and gain muscle at the same time.

Fact #5 – Yes you can. If you're eating good fats, eating a little more protein than your daily protein total, eating all your micronutrients, and doing resistance training, then, when you fast, **your liver will convert your stored fat into glucose to fill the muscles' glycogen stores and shunt the extra protein and micronutrients into the muscle to construct more muscle**.

If you're eating for the checking account (good fats), eating a little more construction material (protein) in your liver's daily income, eating all the construction permits (micronutrients), and moving your liver's property (muscles), then, when you withhold income (fast), your liver will withdraw from its savings account (your stored fat) for glycogen cash (glucose) and send the extra construction material and permits to the property to construct more property (muscle).

Myth #6 – You should eat whole grains.
Fact #6 – **You should not eat whole grains** because for each gram of fiber is about 10 grams of starch, which is **easily converted to stored fat by your liver**.
You should not eat whole grains because they are instant abundant pocket cash for your liver to put directly into its savings account. Fiber is good, starch is bad.

Myth #7 – Dietary carbohydrates are part of a healthy diet.
Fact #7 – **Dietary carbohydrates are part of a failing diet**. If the goal of the diet is to burn fat, then dietary carbohydrates stop you from reaching your goal. If your liver's burning carbs, it's not burning fat.
If the goal of the diet is to force your liver to withdraw from its savings account, then giving your liver a cash income stops your liver from ever withdrawing from its savings account. If your liver is using cash, it's not using its checking or savings account.

Myth #8 – You need dietary carbohydrates to build muscle.

Fact #8 – **You need glucose in your muscles' glycogen stores to build muscle**. Without dietary carbohydrates, your liver converts dietary and stored fat into glucose and puts that into the muscles' glycogen stores.

You need cash in your muscles' pockets to build more property. Without a cash income, your liver goes to the ATM, takes out cash, and puts the cash into the muscles' pockets to build more property.

Myth #9 – You need to get more steps.

Fact #9 – You need to get more steps **up an incline**. Yes, steps are good, but incline steps require more energy and muscle usage than regular steps, so you should shoot to get more steps **up an incline** to increase your liver's spending. Stairs are good.

Myth #10 – Running gets you the six-pack.

Fact #10 – **0g carb/day + fasting + abdominal resistance exercises together get you the six-pack**. Yes, running's good, but it can kill your joints and it's not as effective if you're eating carbohydrates. Instead, **go 0g carb/day, fast, and do leg lift and resistance exercises**.

Myth #11 – You need to count your calories.

Fact #11 – **You need to count your grams**. Look, you eat mass (g) not energy (cal), so you should count what you're actually eating. By counting **0g carb/day** and **1g protein per pound of lean body mass per day** you do not need to count calories. Your totals are met.

CHAPTER 11
FREQUENTLY ASKED QUESTIONS

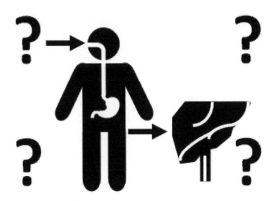

Q: Why can't I lose weight?

A: Rephrase the question to ask, "Why isn't my liver withdrawing from its **savings account (my stored fat)**?" The answer is that your liver sees no need to withdraw from its savings account because its pockets (glycogen stores) are always full of cash (carbs). If your liver's glycogen stores stay full, then there's no need for your liver to burn your stored fat, so stop eating carbs and filling your liver's glycogen stores.

Q: What are you supposed to eat if you completely avoid carbs?

A: **Good fats, lean proteins, and dark leafy green micronutrients** (the logo of the book). No breads, no sugars, no grains, no starches, 0g carb/day.

Q: Won't you lose muscle from completely avoiding carbs?

A: **No**. When your liver is banking correctly and getting enough construction materials (protein) and permits (micronutrients), it not only efficiently uses the checking account (dietary fat) and the savings account (your stored fat) for its energy needs, but **the liver also uses your dietary and stored fat for gluconeogenic muscle glycogen**. Your liver goes to the ATM and extracts the cash it needs from the checking and the savings to pay the muscles' pockets. No dietary carbs needed.

Q: I've been cutting 500 calories a day, but still, I see no weight loss. Why?

A: Because calorie counting doesn't work when you're a carb eater. As a carb eater, if you eat 500 calories fewer per day than you normally eat, then your liver signals the **thyroid to send out hormones that drastically lower your RMR** (the amount of energy your organs use) [17], so what you thought was a 500-calorie deficit for the day now isn't; it might even be a surplus.

When cash eaters reduce their liver's income by 500 calories, their liver contacts the **energy company, the thyroid**, and asks if the energy company can lower the energy bill by putting all the **organs on energy saver mode**. The thyroid then signals all the organs to operate at reduced output, so what you thought was an expensive day for your liver now isn't; your liver might have even netted extra money.

Q: How many carbs should I eat per day?

A: **You need to seriously aim for 0g carb/day**. Your dark leafy green micronutrients will have trace amounts, but that's it.

Q: How much fat should I eat per day?

A: The amount of fat that comes with eating your daily protein total and micronutrient absorption.

Q: How many calories should I eat per day?
A: The amount of calories that comes with eating 1g of protein per pound of lean body mass and absorbing all your micronutrients with a healthy fat per day.

Q: How come some people can burn fat on the traditional carb-based diet?
A: There are two possibilities. One is that those people have **unusually high RMRs** and/or **high levels of amylase**, so their dietary carbs, particularly starches, are efficiently digested and metabolized by the body [16] and the glycogen stores are depleted by the high RMR/total energy expenditure per day [11]. The other reason is that they are an elite athlete and, after burning 4,000 calories per day, they eventually deplete the liver's glycogen stores whether their RMR or levels of amylase are high or not. Both examples are rare unfortunately.

Q: Why do some people lose muscle when they fast?
A: Because they are cash (carb) eaters and they aren't eating anywhere near enough construction materials (protein) or permits (micronutrients) before their extended fast, so, when their liver's pockets (glycogen stores) get empty, the liver panics and attempts to liquidate property (muscle) and its construction materials (protein) for quick pocket cash (glucose).

Q: What do I eat if I've reached my daily protein and micronutrient total and I'm still hungry?

A: An avocado. Cut it open, get a spoon, and eat it. Or you can pair a healthy fat with dark leafy green micronutrients and eat that salad.

Q: What do I do when I'm fasting, but I'm super hungry?

A: Eat an avocado or dark leafy green micronutrient paired with a healthy fat and continue your fast.

Q: Should I eat fruits?

A: What are you eating them for? If the answer is micronutrients, then the only fruit you should ever eat is the **avocado** because it has nearly all the micronutrients and it's essentially no carb. The other fruits simply have too many carbs and not enough micronutrients to be worth eating. **You can get all your micronutrients with avocado and dark leafy greens**.

Q: Should I eat starchy vegetables?

A: No. **Avoid starch in any form**. Any fiber or micronutrient benefit you'd get from starchy vegetables can be achieved with avocado and dark leafy greens, so no starch is needed.

Q: Should I eat beans?

A: Everyone thinks beans are so good for their fiber content, but beans are just a bunch of starch. For each gram of fiber there's two grams of starch. **Avoid starch in any form**.

Q: How do some carb eaters manage to get their liver to burn stored fat?

A: First, these types of people are very rare, but they deplete their liver's glycogen stores with intense exercise and have a naturally high RMR, so briefly their livers become "metabolically flexible" and access some dietary and some stored fat when the glycogen stores deplete. As soon as carbs are reintroduced though, their liver can easily fill its glycogens stores, convert the extra carbs to stored fat, and continue only burning carbs for energy.

Basically, this type of cash eater's liver knows how to write a one-time check but isn't regularly banking and doesn't have a check card. Once the cash eater eats cash again, the liver easily fills its pockets, sends the extra cash to the savings account, and continues only using its pocket cash income for money.

CHAPTER 12
CASH TO CARD MEAL CONVERSIONS

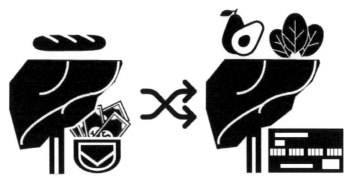

Your liver deserves the best income. These are cash to card conversions to get you ready for banking with your liver.

1. bread/wraps/buns → spinach/kale
2. rice/beans → broccoli/avocado
3. bagel/oatmeal/cereal → eggs
4. pancakes/waffles → bacon/sausage (pig/turkey)
5. table sugar → heavy cream
6. milk → unsweetened almond milk
7. pasta → spinach/asparagus
8. soda/juice → seltzer water/water
9. sweet tea/sweet coffee → unsweetened tea/0g carb cream in coffee/black coffee
10. chips/pretzels/popcorn → 0g carb jerky/pork rinds/almonds
11. french fries/mashed potatoes/hashbrowns → guacamole
12. ketchup/tomato sauce/bbq sauce → olive oil/vinegar
13. cookies/cakes/desserts/treats → almonds/peanuts/seeds
14. ice cream → 0g added sugar chilled peanut/almond butter

CHAPTER 13
TL;DR

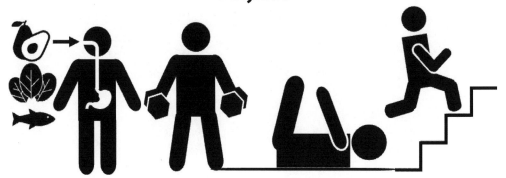

We live in a time where if people have to read too much they shut down, so if the book was **too long** and you **didn't read** it:

1. Eat 0g carbohydrates/day, eat 1g of protein per pound of lean body mass/day, and eat 3-5 cups of dark leafy green micronutrients/day paired with avocado or olive oil.
2. You can fast for 24 hours after regularly doing #1.
3. 2-3 times a week get free weights and do 30 squats, 30 flies, and 30 curls to presses.
4. 2-3 times a week get in leg lift position and do 30 leg lift crunches, 30 starfishes, and 30 ladder climbs.
5. 2-3 times a week find inclines and jog/powerwalk up and down the inclines for at least 15 minutes.
6. Happily live your life without dietary carbohydrates because **dietary carbohydrates are not essential, they're the reason for your extra stored body fat, and they are detrimental to your health.**

REFERENCES

1. Trefts E, Gannon M, Wasserman DH. The liver. *Curr Biol.* 2017;27(21):R1147–R1151. doi: 10.1016/j.cub.2017.09.019. [PMC free article] [PubMed] [CrossRef] [Google Scholar]

2. Ameer F, Scandiuzzi L, Hasnain S, Kalbacher H, Zaidi N. De novo lipogenesis in health and disease. *Metabolism.* 2014;63:895–902. doi: 10.1016/j.metabol.2014.04.003. [PubMed] [CrossRef] [Google Scholar]

3. Pradhan G, Samson SL, Sun Y. Ghrelin: Much More Than a Hunger Hormone. *Curr Opin Clin Nutr Metab Care* (2013) 16(6):619–24. doi: 10.1097/MCO.0b013e328365b9be [PMC free article] [PubMed] [CrossRef] [Google Scholar]

4. Tondt J, Yancy WS, Westman EC. Application of nutrient essentiality criteria to dietary carbohydrates. Nutr Res Rev. 2020 Dec;33(2):260-270. doi: 10.1017/S0954422420000050. Epub 2020 Feb 27. PMID: 32102704.

5. Masood W, Annamaraju P, Uppaluri KR. Ketogenic Diet. In: StatPearls. StatPearls Publishing, Treasure Island (FL); 2021. PMID: 29763005.

6. Puchalska P, Crawford PA. Multi-dimensional roles of ketone bodies in fuel metabolism, signaling, and therapeutics. *Cell Metab.* 2017;**25**:262–284. doi: 10.1016/j.cmet.2016.12.022. [PMC free article] [PubMed] [CrossRef] [Google Scholar]

7. Zhang X, Yang S, Chen J, Su Z. Unraveling the Regulation of Hepatic Gluconeogenesis. Front Endocrinol (Lausanne). 2018;9:802. [PMC free article] [PubMed]

8. Alves-Bezerra M, Cohen DE. Triglyceride Metabolism in the Liver. *Compr Physiol.* 2017;8(1):1–8. Epub 2018/01/23. doi: 10.1002/cphy.c170012 ; PubMed Central PMCID: PMC6376873. [PMC free article] [PubMed] [CrossRef] [Google Scholar]

9. Frandsen J., Poggi A.I., Ritz C., Larsen S., Dela F., Helge J.W. Peak fat oxidation rate is closely associated with plasma free fatty acid concentrations in women; similar to men. *Front. Physiol.* 2021;12:696261. doi: 10.3389/fphys.2021.696261. [PMC free article] [PubMed] [CrossRef] [Google Scholar]

10. Van Dijk M., Dijk F.J., Hartog A., van Norren K., Verlaan S., van Helvoort A., Jaspers R.T., Luiking Y. Reduced Dietary Intake of Micronutrients with Antioxidant Properties Negatively Impacts Muscle Health in Aged Mice: Reduced Dietary Intake of Micronutrients. *J. Cachexia Sarcopenia Muscle.* 2018;9:146–159. doi: 10.1002/jcsm.12237. [PMC free article] [PubMed] [CrossRef] [Google Scholar]

11. McMurray RG, Soares J, Caspersen CJ, McCurdy T. Examining variations of resting metabolic rate of adults: a public health perspective. *Med Sci Sports Exerc.* 2014;**46**(7):1352. [PMC free article] [PubMed] [Google Scholar]

12. Antunes, M.M. , Godoy, G. , de Almeida-Souza, C.B. , da Rocha, B.A. , da Silva-Santi, L.G. , Masi, L.N. , Carbonera, F. , Visentainer, J.V. *et al.* (2020) A high-carbohydrate diet induces greater inflammation than a high-fat diet in mouse skeletal muscle. Brazilian J. Med. *Biol Res* 53.e9039 [PMC free article] [PubMed] [Google Scholar]

13. Lintermans LL, Stegeman CA, Heeringa P, Abdulahad WH. T cells in vascular inflammatory diseases. *Front Immunol.* 2014;5:504. [PMC free article] [PubMed] [Google Scholar]

14. Ludwig D.S., Hu F.B., Tappy L., Brand-Miller J. Dietary Carbohydrates: Role of Quality and Quantity in Chronic Disease. *BMJ.* 2018;361:k2340. doi: 10.1136/bmj.k2340. [PMC free article] [PubMed] [CrossRef] [Google Scholar]

15. Wheeler M.L., Dunbar S.A., Jaacks L.M., Wahida K., Mayer-Davis E.J., Judith W.R., Jr., William S. Macronutrients, Food Groups, and Eating Patterns in the Management of Diabetes. *Diabet. Care.* 2010;35:434–445. doi: 10.2337/dc11-2216. [PMC free article] [PubMed] [CrossRef] [Google Scholar]

16. Peyrot des Gachons C., Breslin P.A.S. Salivary Amylase: Digestion and Metabolic Syndrome. *Curr. Diabetes Rep.* 2016;16:102. doi: 10.1007/s11892-016-0794-7. [PMC free article] [PubMed] [CrossRef] [Google Scholar]

17. Mullur R., Liu Y.-Y., Brent G.A. Thyroid hormone regulation of metabolism. *Physiol. Rev.* 2014;94:355–382. doi: 10.1152/physrev.00030.2013. [PMC free article] [PubMed] [CrossRef] [Google Scholar]

18. Barclay AW, Petocz P, McMillan-Price J, Flood VM, Prvan T, Mitchell P, Brand-Miller JC. Glycemic index, glycemic load, and chronic disease risk--a meta-analysis of observational studies. Am J Clin Nutr. 2008 Mar;87(3):627-37. doi: 10.1093/ajcn/87.3.627. PMID: 18326601.

19. Kim Y., Chen J., Wirth M.D., Shivappa N., Hebert J.R. Lower dietary inflammatory index scores are associated with lower glycemic index scores among college students. *Nutrients.* 2018;10:182. doi: 10.3390/nu10020182.
[PMC free article] [PubMed] [CrossRef] [Google Scholar]

20. Kersten S. Mechanisms of nutritional and hormonal regulation of lipogenesis. *EMBO Rep.* 2001;2(4):282–6. doi: 10.1093/embo-reports/kve071
[PMC free article] [PubMed] [CrossRef] [Google Scholar]

21. Layman DK, Evans E, Baum JI, Seyler J, Erickson DJ, Boileau RA. Dietary protein and exercise have additive effects on body composition during weight loss in adult women. *J Nutr.* 2005;**135**:1903–10.
[PubMed] [Google Scholar]

IMAGES USED

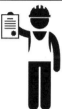

1. "Worker Permit" by Gan Khoon Lay, from Noun Project
https://thenounproject.com/icon/worker-permit-1585647/

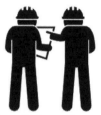

2. "Construction Planning" by Gan Khoon Lay, from Noun Project
https://thenounproject.com/icon/construction-planning-2751747/

3. "Cheese" by Shirley Wu, from Noun Project
https://thenounproject.com/icon/cheese-12092/

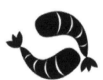

4. "Shrimp" by Winn Creative, from Noun Project
https://thenounproject.com/icon/shrimp-1651512/

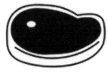

5. "Beef" by Pedro Bonfim, from Noun Project
https://thenounproject.com/icon/beef-4514803/

6. "Spinach" by Phạm Thanh Lộc, from Noun Project
https://thenounproject.com/icon/spinach-2710074/

7. "Asparagus" by Phạm Thanh Lộc, from Noun Project
https://thenounproject.com/icon/asparagus-2710029/

8. "Cabbage" by Andika Julian, from Noun Project
https://thenounproject.com/icon/cabbage-4405438/

9. "Kale" by Amethyst Studio, from Noun Project
https://thenounproject.com/icon/kale-4130639/

10.   "Broccoli" by Nathan Stang, from Noun Project
https://thenounproject.com/icon/broccoli-26078/

11.   "Brussel Sprouts" by Laymik, from Noun Project
https://thenounproject.com/icon/brussel-sprouts-436996/

12.   "Romaine" by Monkik, from Noun Project
https://thenounproject.com/icon/romaine-3382334/

13.   "Almond" by Parashanth Rapolu, from Noun Project
https://thenounproject.com/icon/almond-2070165/

14.   "Bacon" by Ji Sub Jeong, from Noun Project
https://thenounproject.com/icon/bacon-93671/

15.	"Sausage" by unknown, from Noun Project
https://thenounproject.com/browse/icons/term/sausage

NOTICE

All other images that appear in this book, but were not listed in "Images Used", were created by the author, Micah Frye, and any use of those images requires written permission.
mfrye1@gmail.com

ABOUT THE AUTHOR

Micah Frye, residing in the suburbs of Baltimore, is a first-time author who, through years of watching and experiencing people's metabolic struggles, has decided it's time to erase our flawed knowledge of diet and metabolism. Though a full-time high school teacher, husband, and dad, when Micah isn't coaching wrestling, he finds time to research and show simplified ways to understand complicated scientific concepts to his children, students, and wrestlers. Micah has gone from nearly 30% body fat to 8% body fat simply by banking with his liver. Stop eating cash and start banking with your liver.

You can contact Micah Frye: mfrye1@gmail.com with the subject "Banking With Your Liver"

Printed in Great Britain
by Amazon

86810745R00034